WEIGHT LOSS: A STRATEGIC AND HEALTHY APPROACH TO STAY FIT AND SLIM FOR LIFE

LONG TERM BENEFITS OF HEALTHY WEIGHT LOSS MANAGEMENT

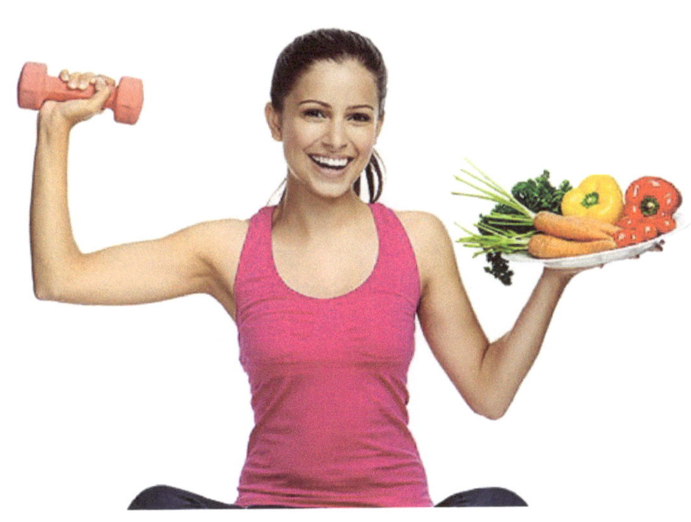

Table of Contents

INTRODUCTION

In reality, there is only one true effective way to get rid of fat and decrease your body weight. That is by moving more and eating less through a regimen of diet and exercise.

Many people shudder at the word diet, and needlessly so. You can condition your body to accept a certain lifestyle, a smarter (and still fun) lifestyle. Our bodies are extremely adaptable to our environment and will adjust to the changes we make in a rather short period.

Instituting a new diet regimen and psychologically forcing your body to adapt to the new environment is a very effective way to accomplish permanent fat loss and a healthier body.

Once you decide to lose weight and, specifically, are determined to decrease your body's fat content, it is best to not go cold turkey cutting out all calories at once. Rather set short-term goals to accomplish your ultimate weight and fitness goal.

For instance, you could choose to cut your sugar intake by half for the first week or two, and then gradually cut out all refined sugar in the third week or by the end of the month.

Another idea is to start doing minor increases in exercises, such as walking, in the first week. Try walking an extra block or two and then increase that amount a little each week.

In this respect, you are not running a marathon the first week, rather gradually building up to a substantial change in your amount of exercise over the course of several weeks.

In order to effectively increase your fat loss, it is very helpful to make specific, small weekly plans on what you want to accomplish. In other words, you could decide to lose 2 pounds in the first week and then one pound each week after that, instead of saying "I'm going to lose 20 pounds sometime soon."

You will find that by making small goals and working slowly toward your ultimate end of decreasing your weight and increasing your fat loss, you will more easily meet your goal. Consistent, small changes are easier for the body than one big change that does not last.

Remember, it took time for you to gain weight and it will take time to lose it. The real weight loss programs that work are not those that will help you "shed 20 pounds in a week or increase your fat loss over night."

Real weight loss programs require determination and adjustments to your body through a change in mindset and lifestyle environment. Through smart changes in diet and exercise, you will see of fat loss you desire.

This book will help you understand how to stay fit with healthy weight loss in almost all ways.

Happy Reading!

CHAPTER 1
WHAT IS WEIGHT LOSS?

Weight-loss typically involves the loss of fat, water and muscle. Weight management is about long-term success and will hopefully last a lifetime. Weight gain is often linked to certain medication, such as HRT, the contraceptive pill and steroids.

What Is Weight Loss?

Weight loss is attempting to lower your total body weight. It simply refers to a lower number on a scale. Your body weight is composed of all the parts of your body such as muscles, fat, bones, water, organs, tissues, blood, water etc. When you lose weight, you lose a little bit of... fat, muscle and water.

You lose fat... but very little and along with the fat you lose muscle and some amount of water. The higher you reduce your calorie intake, the faster you drop weight and the more muscle mass you lose. Loss of muscle affects your health and your overall appearance.

When you lose weight too quickly, your body cannot maintain its muscle. Because muscle requires more calories to sustain itself, your body begins to metabolize it so that it can reserve the incoming calories for its survival.

It protects its fat stores as a defense mechanism to ensure your survival in case of future famine and instead use lean tissue or muscle to provide it with calories it needs to keep its vital organs such as your brain, heart, kidneys and liver functioning. If you reach a point where you have very little fat or muscle, your body will metabolize your organs to keep your brain functioning leading to heart attack, stroke and liver and kidney failure.

As the body loses more muscle mass, the body's overall metabolic rate decreases. The metabolic rate is the rate at which the body burns calories and is partly determined by the amount of muscle you have.

So the more muscle you have, the higher your metabolic rate; the less muscle you have, the lower your metabolic rate and fewer calories you burn. This explains why it is crucial to protect your metabolic rate and not have muscle loss.

Loss of muscle also leads to loss of tone underneath the skin leaving you soft and unshapely with no form or contour. If you lose weight too rapidly, your skin won't have time to adjust either. Also, muscle is what gives you strength and loss of it means a weak body.

With weight loss you shrink in size and become a smaller version of yourself with a fragile frame with saggy skin.

Weight loss works in the short run to make you smaller but is temporary. Almost everyone rebounds and regains the weight. This forces you to find another diet. And then another one, and another one - because eventually they'll all fail.

CHAPTER 2
A STRATEGIC APPROACH TO GETTING SLIM FOR LIFE

The first step to permanent, healthy weight loss is to learn to love yourself. Yes, you read that right! Getting yourself into the right frame of mind and allowing yourself to be loved -- by others, but most of all by yourself are the best way to make lasting change for the better.

The reason you're overweight now is because of self-sabotaging thoughts which prevent you from truly being the person you deserve to be. Most overweight people just don't know how to think like a slim person.

We all have a background conversation going on in our minds, constantly affecting the way we're feeling and affecting our behavior. It's frequently negative and outdated, and when we're not consciously aware of it, we can't do anything to change it.

With the power of our unconscious thoughts on our side, we can actually get to where we want to be and this means healthy weight loss without massive effort. Learn to catch your negative chatter and turn it around to the positive.

Stop comparing yourself to other people. You are you, and you're great as you are, even before you lose the weight. You're lovable, attractive and unique. Please don't forget that! And don't focus on how "unfair" it is that other people seem to eat whatever they want and not gain weight. Most slim people restrict their eating to some extent, whether they're aware of it or not.

To gain the slim body you desire, you also need to love your body just the way it is. Not as it will be once you reach your optimal weight, but as it is right now. This is the way to literally "think yourself slim". Appreciate the fact that you have a strong, lovely body, and know that it's embarking on a journey towards full health and wellness.

Now, see if you can start to recognize the difference between genuine hunger (a feeling in your stomach) and other triggers. Many overweight people eat for emotional reasons, and just push their feelings down with food. If this is you, learn to see that, however much you eat, this won't take the emotion away.

If you are hungry, by all means eat something. You're starting to listen to what your body is actually telling you. Eat little and reasonably often, but never go beyond the feeling of just having satisfied the hunger. Over-eating isn't just bad for you, it's uncomfortable too.

Don't deny yourself any particular foods, however calorie-laden. But if it's an unhealthy option, just eat a little of it and throw the rest away or keep it for another day.

Healthy weight loss doesn't mean existing purely on lettuce and cottage cheese. Rather, it means being in control of what you choose to eat. You may decide to eat a small slice of cake on one day, but then you could up your vegetable intake the next day, knowing that your body is loving you for it.

Think of how it'll feel when you feel like wearing sexy, fitted clothes again, when your tread becomes lighter, and when you start getting compliments on your new slim look!

CHAPTER 3
LONG TERM BENEFITS OF HEALTHY WEIGHT LOSS

You will always hear such general benefits as looking better, feeling better, better self-esteem, sexier, easier to climb stairs, and so on. But what are some of the very real reasons that people might really need to be thinking of?

Here are a few short term and long term benefits of a good weight loss program.

1. Several major causes of death, including hypertension, heart disease, and strokes can be avoided or prevented by weight loss.

Heart disease and stroke are two of the major causes of death and disability in both men and women in America. High cholesterol, which can contribute to heart disease, tends to be more prevalent in overweight people. Death from heart disease and stroke often strikes without warning yet could be prevented by a program of regular exercise and sensible nutrition.

The weight loss does not have to be great, either. Minor decreases in weight can significantly decrease the chance of developing heart disease or having a stroke. Of course, when we speak of "weight loss" we really ought to be saying "fat loss". It is not the weight which is the issue as much as it is the quantity of excess fat which has accumulated in the body.

2. Healthy weight loss can help prevent Type II diabetes.

Diabetes, like many other problems not only puts you in danger of death, but also changes the manner in which you can live your life. Type I and Type II diabetes have been linked to being overweight.

It has been shown that, in addition to helping prevent diabetes, regular exercise and healthy nutrition can help reduce the effects of diabetes and perhaps reduce the dependency on treatments, such as insulin.

It doesn't take much. Change a few habits, cut out the wrong kinds of food, or substitute the right ones, take some regular walks to help burn fat, and you are on your way.

3. Weight loss helps reduce the risk of cancer.

Many types of cancer, such as breast cancer and colon cancer, just to name two, have been linked to being overweight. While carrying extra fat is not the only contributor to the development of cancer, it has been shown that shedding that extra fat can be an important factor in preventing the development of cancer.

Some other cancers which seem to be linked to obesity in this way are cancer of the uterus, gallbladder, ovary, prostate, and rectum.

4. Weight loss helps ease the pains of arthritis.

This is particularly true of osteoarthritis. When you are overweight, the fat you carry tends to push joints out of alignment, and the excess weight produces extra stress on joints. This can contribute to the development and discomfort of arthritis. Regular exercise can also help keep joints strong, flexible, and well lubricated.

5. Weight loss can improve your sleep.

One common problem associated with being overweight is sleep apnea. In this condition, you temporarily stop breathing for brief periods. There is generally also heavy breathing and snoring all of which interferes with getting a good night's sleep and rest.

This leads to tiredness and drowsiness during the day. Many people have found that losing even a few pounds can help head off this problem. Additionally, regular exercise and proper nutrition can contribute to more restful sleep and fewer problems related to stress and fatigue.

CHAPTER 4
HOW TO BEGIN YOUR DIET FOR LOSING WEIGHT?

Cut Back Your Fat and Sugar Intake

First thing to consider is to apply the combination of eating healthy and at the same time curtailing your fat and sugar intake. More importantly, you should be physically active. An effective exercise routine should be part of your weight loss plan.

If you've been inclined on eating sugary and fatty junk foods and have limited physical activity, you basically need a change of lifestyle so that you will lose weight. Not that you have to do it drastically. Healthy weight loss needs you to adjust your healthy eating plan gradually. If you force and do it abruptly, dieting could be hard on your body.

Likewise don't be too keen to overwhelm your body with heavy exercises at the beginning. Don't be so hasty in running a marathon if you've had zero exercise in the first place. In your diet and exercise plan to lose weight, take time to commence with it one baby step to the next at a time.

How to begin your diet for losing weight?

Make a start by stopping your weight gain. That is, you should stop gaining weight first. Be careful with the foods that you eat. Restrict your consumption of sugars and fats. The best diet for weight loss includes a balanced diet.

Take note that numerous fad diets do not fall into the category of balanced diets at all. Some of them would re□uire you to eat too much of one nutrient, such as protein while skipping another important food group such as whole grains. Often, fad diets also cut out dairy foods in your meals. These diets are not filling and healthy.

Eat A Healthy And Balanced Diet - Change Your Lifestyle

Vegetables are part of a healthy diet and eating them will make you lose weight. However, see to it that your vegetable consumption can be a sustained eating habit and lifestyle.

For a balanced diet to burn calories and shed pounds, prepare 3 servings of fruits and veggies, 2 servings of dairy foods (at least), 1 or 2 portions of meat and nuts and seeds for your meals.

In the process of losing weight, detoxify your body. Cut out your intake of fatty and sugary foods. While doing so after some time, you'll notice that you'll get rid and get used to skipping sweets and fatty foods wherein you'll feel you're as healthy as can be.

Apply The Magic Formula For Weight Loss - Burn Calories

Healthy weight loss is not all about dieting. To optimize your health and fitness program, you have to exercise. The magic formula for fast and healthy weight loss remains, and that is to burn more calories than you eat.

Fifteen minutes of exercise a day is sufficient for an effective health and fitness program. You simply won't lose weight but will feel healthy and energized as well.

Make that decision to lose weight and be healthy. It's a wise decision that will affect the longevity and quality of your life. Adhere to a healthy and balanced diet for weight loss, exercise regularly and limit your consumption of junk food. You'll be healthier and happier and have the zest to succeed in life.

Regardless of what you do in life, it is important to optimize on your performance all the time. This is done through checking on whatever you eat as well as drink such that it does not exceed or go beyond the required limits.

CHAPTER 5
DAILY DIETING IDEAS

So you're in search of some ideas and suggestions for a daily diet plan that not only works, but lasts. I assume you've made the decision to lose some weight and want to make real dietary changes to your life.

I will share with you simple and delicious meal ideas that are not only guaranteed to help you lose weight, but to keep you full and satisfied throughout your day. It's my hope that at the end of reading this chapter, you'll have the knowledge and confidence to create your own diet plan.

But first, let me explain a little about understanding calories and how to workout your daily allowance for speedy weight loss.

Calories: A good way to understand calories is to think of them as energy. A person becomes overweight usually because they consume more energy (food & drink) than they use up through exercise during the day. This is such a simple way of looking at it. But although most people know this, many believe that they are just big boned or heavy set.

So being honest with yourself is the first step, no excuses. Although metabolism can have a small part to play, your physical body that you see before you is the result of this energy imbalance. To lose weight you must eat less calories than your daily recommendation until you reach your goal weight. Simple right?

The average woman needs around 2,000 calories a day. The average man needs 2,500 calories. To lose weight you must consume 500 calories less each day. So it's very important to get used to reading food labels and writing down your calorie amount.

Breakfast: This is commonly thought of as the most important meal of the day, for good reason. Your brain expects to be refueled several times a day, otherwise it can't function at its full capacity.

A healthy breakfast can provide some of the vitamins and minerals you need for good health. By skipping breakfast, your also more likely to be hungry and over eat later in the day.

If breakfast cereal is your thing, choose a wholegrain variety instead of the many sugar-coated cereals on the market. Fresh or dried fruits add a sweet hint instead of sugar, and only use skimmed milk or fat-free yoghurt.

Wholemeal and wholegrain toast or bagels with a low-fat spread is a ☐uick and healthy way to start the day. These contain B vitamins, vitamin E and lots of fiber, which keeps you fuller for longer. White breads also contain a range of vitamins and minerals, but has less fiber and is sometimes higher in calories.

Eggs are a great choice as part of a healthy breakfast. They are high in minerals and vitamins and are a fantastic source of protein. Try eggs, grilled tomatoes and mushrooms on a wholegrain bagel or a slice of toast. With a crack of fresh black pepper, this breakfast will certainly set you up for the day and keep you satisfied till lunch.

Lunch and evening meal: Try to space out your breakfast, lunch and evening meal as equally apart as you can. They do say to eat before 6pm in the evening, but in my experience, this is not essential as long as you eat within at least 2 hours before bed if you can.

The key to a successful diet plan is to never be hungry. Studies show that eating small amounts more often (5 to 6 times a day) is much more effective than eating 3 large meals. In between your 3 main meals, get in the habit of snacking on fruit and low calorie foods, staying within your daily calorie allowance.

For lunch and evening meal, try to experiment with flavors as often as possible. This is a good way of getting away from boring, bland and unexciting plates of food. Don't be afraid to spice up your cooking and try new things.

Choose lean cuts of meat, chicken and fish and try marinading them for a few hours before cooking, although this is not essential. Most marinades and rubs are not fattening, but if any recipes you find are □uite high in calorie, then you can always tweak them to suit you. Here are some low fat, simple marinades to get you started...

Garlic, mustard marinade: Easy yet delicious. This works best with chicken, pork and beef. Simply mix all ingredients together and coat the meat.

1 Clove garlic, crushed

1 tablespoons Dijon mustard (or any other mustard if preferred)

1 teaspoons thyme (optional)

Spicy Indian marinade: This is definitely one for the barbecue or simply baked in the oven. Perfect for chicken, lamb and firm white fish such as cod or monkfish.

4 tablespoons low-fat natural yoghurt

1 clove garlic crushed

1 inch fresh root ginger, peeled, finely grated

Juice of half lemon

1 teaspoon ground turmeric

2 green cardamom pods, lightly crushed

1 teaspoon ground cumin

1 teaspoon ground coriander

Pinch of salt

For your long term health, make sure the diet is based on sound principles that have proven to result in both fat loss and overall health. If you lose too much, too fast, you'll just be setting yourself up for failure.

The following should give you some guidelines on choosing a plan that works for you. Remember that fads come and go, but effective fat loss principles basically stay the same.

The first step in planning your diet is to determine the number of calories you consume on a daily basis. How do you figure that out? The best thing to do is to get a calorie counter that has a database of foods and a lookup feature.

After every meal or snack, you log what you've eaten or had to drink and the calorie counter will calculate the totals for you. Of course, you can always just use a pencil and paper and tally up the results yourself.

You should count your calories for about a week to get a good idea of the average number of daily calories you're consuming. Calorie counting seems to have a powerful psychological effect as well. It will make you think twice about eating that extra dessert or serving of fries if you have to add it to your score.

The next step will be to determine the number of calories you need to maintain your present weight. For this purpose, you can use a Resting Metabolic Rate Calculator.

To lose weight, you need to start eating fewer calories than your maintenance level. The recommended amount of calories to cut out for effective weight loss is between 15-20% of the daily maintenance level.

Cutting out more than 20% of your maintenance level calories is not recommended for any quick fat loss diet. Doing so will only slow down your metabolism, which means you'll burn fewer calories.

When following a quick fat loss diet, it's important to ensure that you're meeting your nutritional needs. You can't just consume empty calories from refined sources like sugar or starchy foods. Your calories need to come from fresh fruits and vegetables, whole grains, low fat dairy products and lean meat.

The optimal balance would be to get 45% of your calories from carbohydrates, 35% from lean protein sources and 20% from healthy fat sources.

Eating breakfast, lunch and dinner won't work for a quick fat loss diet. You will need to eat smaller amounts more frequently, perhaps 5-7 smaller meals per day. That means eating every 2 to 3 hours throughout the day.

CHAPTER 6
HEALTHY OPTIONS WHEN EATING OUT

Sticking to a low-fat diet can be difficult, especially when dining out and going to parties with friends who might unintentionally pressure you into eating high calorie/fatty foods.

You feel you have no control over what you can eat and often feel awkward at the prospect of being seen to be a 'boring person'. It can be done, however, and there are many low-fat tricks for any situation.

Eating outside of the house, beyond your sphere of control, can be tough; especially when quantity is deemed more important than quality. In times when money is tight everyone feels that they should be getting value for money, but that does not necessarily mean large portions.

The downside to this is you can quite quickly consume a daily calorie allowance in one meal. Further complications exist for people with high cholesterol who need to control their fat intake. Here are a few thoughts:

•Planning ahead always helps when dining out. Most dining out places have a presence on the internet so you can often access websites to see what is on the menu and choose your courses in advance. Choose a reserve as well in case one of your preferred courses have run out or have been changed for a more fatty option.

•Pick your food with words like 'steamed, grilled, poached or boiled' in mind. They tend to be the most low-fat ways of preparing food where quite often lies the bulk of fats we are trying to avoid.

•Avoid "breaded", "lightly breaded" or "battered" foods. Nothing healthy, however nice tasting, comes from food dipped in starch and floating around in a vat of oil or lard.

•Stay away from anything pan-fried or stir-fried, prepared with lots of oil or butter.

•Having the right tools is key to any successful project and this includes eating responsibly. Become accustomed to reasonable portion sizes by investing in digital food scales. It will help you to become accustomed to what 'acceptable portions' look like. Many online retailers sell such scales.

•As a rule of thumb, no serving of food should be bigger than your fist. If it is and you want what you paid for, divide it and ask for a "to go" box and refrigerate it for later.

•Always try and substitute vegetables or salad for French fries. You'll save on fat and calories.

•Don't be tricked by disguised entree salads with fried noodles and/or tons of full salad dressing. Salad dressing and condiments alone can add significant calories and fat that you do not intend to eat.

•Always order salad dressing and any salad toppings on the side. This allows you to control your intake. Start to savour your crunchy vegetables.

•Get your baked potato dry and stay clear of high-fat fillings. Ask for your vegetables steamed.

•Always ask for brown rice instead of white - it's better for you whatever your dietary requirements are.

Not being able to prepare for one's own meals at home should not excuse anybody not to eat nutritious foods. Eating out is always almost tempting. What with barbecue at the neighbor's place and clients to entertain, eating out healthy comes very rare these days.

For this matter, I will provide you 4 ways to keep your food healthy when eating out. Even when you are not adhering to Abs Diet, the following guidelines shall also prove to be helpful.

1. Have a pre-loved food or meal. A few hours before eating out at a restaurant, eat a small snack like a tuna sandwich, protein shake, oatmeal, or even a large meal. This method prevents you from feasting on forbidden foods at the restaurant. It is also helpful in keeping one's blood sugar from rising.

2. Know the nature of foods and their ingredients. Before deciding on which dish to order, try asking how such dishes are prepared. While chicken may be great, certain manners of cooking may pose threats to your weight.

An example of an unhealthy chicken dish is chicken parmesan which is breaded and fried before it is finally baked. Avoid selecting foods that have sauces containing more sodium than how much you should have in a week. Sauce must be ordered on the side to control the Quantity.

3. When you are doubtful, be safe by choosing salad. There are delectable and healthy salads containing grilled chicken, fish, vegetables, or shrimp. Ensure that the cheese, bacon bits, and croutons are limited.

Equally important is the avoidance of sliced meats for most of them are highly processed, unless there is an option for a freshly-baked turkey breast sliced off the bone. Emphasis is also placed on choosing the salad dressing and allowing your fork to dip into it every few bites.

4. Indulge in desserts. Do not spoil the moment by skipping sweets. Order either a cup of coffee or a sherbet.

CHAPTER 7
WHAT MAKES A WEIGHT LOSS EXERCISE EFFECTIVE?

This may seem like a question which is going to lead into a complicated answer, but it really isn't. The key to any efficient fat burning move is the amount of muscles you use per repetition and the level of intensity at which you perform it. Remember your body will also use calories to repair your body for days after you workout when using weights.

To lose weight you need to burn more calories than you consume on a daily basis, simple. Your body burns the most amounts of calories when using its muscles.

So taking this into account, to lose weight in the quickest time you need to be performing exercises that moves over a series of joints and a collection of muscles, if not all of your muscles (Compound exercises).

Below is a list of exercises set into 3 section (Beginner, intermediate, advanced).

Beginner weight loss exercises that are simple and effective

These are the body's basic functional exercises. They teach you how to move through your natural range safely by conditioning your joints and developing the correct motor skills (The way your body moves).

In addition to this, these basic exercises will set you up to progress onto the next stage and leave you with sculptured, toned muscles once the fat is eliminated. As well as using the below weighted exercises you should mix in cardio in the form of continuous training and short interval sprints.

Once you have progressed through to the next stages (intermediate and advance), don't forget to still include the simple exercises as they are still effective weight loss tools. Just increase the weights and intensity by including them in supersets / tri-sets.

• Squat

• Squat and press

- Static lunges

- Dead lift

- Dead lift curl

- Dead lift curl and press

- Press up

- Dumbbell swing

- Burpee

Intermediate weight loss exercises

Developing on from your basic level, these set of movements become more dynamic. By doing this we are placing our muscles into greater stress which will result in increased muscle definition. Furthermore it will take your fitness and endurance to the next step.

To get the most out of your weight loss programme you should start adding supersets (Performing two exercises one after each other) and increase your interval sprints. This will ensure that you maintain your progress.

- S□uat and row (cables)

- Alternate dumbbell swing

- Alternate lunges

- Walking lunges

- Burpee variations

- Dumbbell snatch

- Dumbbell clean and jerk

- Cross body snatch

- Weighted ski

Advanced weight loss exercises

Now you're at the stage where your fitness and endurance should be at a high level and you can perform supersets and sprints efficiently, with a level of ease.

Taking this into consideration we need to raise the bar again by including Tri-sets (performing 3 exercises continuously one after each other). This will get your lungs burning and really test your stamina. Obviously with such an intensive workout the fat will drop of you.

• Burpee Variations with equipment

• Alternate dumbbell clean and jerk

• Alternate dumbbell snatch

• Plyometric jump variations

• Pull ups

• Dips

Don't forget you should mix and match all the exercises through the levels above to maintain a constant weight loss and making sure that your body doesn't adapt to your training. If your body does adapt to your training it will result in a reduced fat burn, so keep on your toes and vary your routines.

CHAPTER 8
SUPER FOODS FOR WEIGHT LOSS

These natural foods go beyond the 'common' variety as they are rich in phytochemicals and antioxidants which slow down the aging process and help your body lose weight.

Here are the best foods for weight loss and why they provide everything you need for optimal health.

1. Blueberries

These yummy little berries are rich in antioxidants. Also full of flavonoids and proanthocyandins they help protect memory and cognition. A popular addition to any fat loss program, they taste great whipped up in a low-fat smoothie, used in whole-wheat pancakes or muffins or just to add a new dimension to your fruit salad.

2. Broccoli

Broccoli has an abundance of health boosting properties. It contains isothiocyanantes which stimulates the body's production of cancer fighting enzymes. It has as much calcium as a glass of milk and more vitamin C than an orange.

In addition, it is one of the richest sources of vitamin A in any fruit or vegetable. The only catch is you do need to eat it raw to benefit from all this goodness. If you cannot handle it raw, then just lightly steam before tossing through a salad or stirring through whole-wheat noodles.

3. Ginger

Used throughout history for medicinal purposes, ginger helps protect against cancer as well as boosting the immune system. It helps fight infection in our body, increases digestive enzyme activity and is one of the natural weight loss foods that speed up the metabolism and burn fat.

Ginger is also a popular remedy for nausea, making it a safe natural choice for pregnant women. Sip hot ginger tea with a drizzle of honey, use in Asian stir fries and grate a little through healthy marinades and sauces.

4. Linseeds

Linseeds contain the essential omega 3 fatty acids which reduce cholesterol. Not only do they have anti-cancer properties but they also can help manage menopausal symptoms.

They are good for bowel health and soothe digestion. Just a tablespoon of linseeds a day will give you the omega 3 fats that you require. Sprinkle them over your cereal or stir through soups and casseroles. Linseeds should be stored in the fridge.

5. Oats

Containing large amount of soluble fibre, oats help lower cholesterol levels and improve bowel health. They have a low GI (glycaemic index) which means they make the perfect breakfast to supercharge your day. Oats are a popular recommendation in most weight loss programs.

6. Salmon

A fantastic source of omega 3 fats, protein and vitamin D. Healthy fat loss programs recommend eating salmon twice a week, as it reduces triglyceride levels.

Any leftover calories that your body does not burn are turned into triglycerides, which are a type of fat. Poach or grill salmon, and serve with a leafy salad or steamed vegetables. Combine tinned salmon with mashed sweet potatoes to make healthy patties - kids also love them.

7. Soy

Soy protein contains antioxidant isoflavones which counteract the buildup of cholesterol in blood vessels, reducing the risk of heart attack and blood clots. It is also great for bone health and preventing osteoporosis.

Make sure you choose soy products that are not genetically modified. Use soy protein or tofu instead of burgers and chicken in recipes. Enjoy soy milk over your cereal or in tasty fruit smoothies.

8. Tea

Numerous studies have shown that the powerful antioxidant polyphenols in tea reduce the risk of cancers and also lower cholesterol levels. In addition, drinking tea helps lower the stress hormone cortisol.

Green tea in particular has had much discussion regarding its weight loss benefits. Actually all teas contain polyphenols and therefore all have positive benefits. Ideally, drink your tea without milk to receive the most benefit.

9. Tomatoes

Tomatoes, which are low in calories, are a versatile health conscious ingredient for any weight loss program. Just add tomatoes to your pasta sauce to boost your antioxidant intake and to lower your risk of chronic diseases, particularly prostate cancer. They are rich in lycopene, which fights damaging free radicals and also high in vitamin C.

There are so many exciting ways you incorporate tomatoes into your meals. Whether it be pureed into sauces, chopped through summer salads or thrown into a whole-wheat tortilla, this fabulous super food is a must.

10. Yogurt

Yogurt is a favorite with many dieters. Not only does its creamy texture help satisfy cravings, it is also a great source of calcium, protein, vitamin B12 and riboflavin. What is more it contains probiotics which promote a healthy gut and protect the immune system.

Use sugar free, low fat yogurt as a substitute for cream in sauces, curries, and desserts. It is fantastic as a 'quick snack' on the run and can be cooked in both savoury and sweet recipes.

What you don't know, though, is that you are exposed to other types of foods that may deceptively look fine to eat but in reality contain a lot of fat and calories. To help you along your road to fitness, take note of the following types of food to avoid for weight loss.

Rice Cakes

Rice, in general, has a very high glycemic index, which means that when you eat them, it highly affects your blood glucose levels. Simple carbohydrates of this type can stimulate fat storage as well as slow down how fast your body burns up fat.

It's the food to avoid for weight loss because it tricks your body into wanting more once you've had it. So, when you try and cut back on it, you feel more intense cravings for it.

Fruit Juice

Fruit juice, at least the commercially-prepared ones, are calorie-dense and have lots of sugar. You might get tricked into thinking that they are healthy because they have fruit. It's better to say actually that they have fruit flavors. Drinking commercially-prepared fruit juices is just like drinking sugared water.

They're the food to avoid for weight loss because it taste good but they don't do anything good for your health. By replacing commercially-prepared fruit juices with water, you can save as much as 200 calories for every cup as well as significantly cutting back on your intake of sugar.

Flavored Oatmeal

Oatmeal is used in a lot of nutritional plans. However, sugar ranks quite high in the ingredients list of your favorite flavored oatmeal. This makes it, yes, an excellent source of fiber but sadly, also of lots of sugar.

If you absolutely must have your oatmeal, try sticking with unflavored oatmeal and use non-fat milk and fruits to add flavor to it. Not only will you get your fiber but you also satisfy a portion of your calcium and fruit needs for the day.

Alcohol

While not necessarily containing a lot of fat, alcohol does contain a lot of calories on its own. And by the time you add all the mixers in--sodas, juices, and others--you're already packing in a lot calories in one glass or shot.

As if that's not a problem enough, excessive amounts of alcohol in your body actually interferes with its ability to metabolize nutrients, most especially protein. This means that it affects your body's ability of building muscle.

And if you don't know, building muscle helps speed up the fat-burning processes in your body. Alcohol then, in excessive amounts, is one type of food to avoid for weight loss.

Salad Dressing

Salads make excellent food choices to help you achieve your weight loss goals. However, they become less-than-good choices when you decide to add those fattening salad dressings.

Your regular salad dressing has about between 6 to 8 grams of fat so that's about 75 calories for every teaspoon. If you normally put about 3 or 4 teaspoons of salad dressing unto your salad, you're adding as much as 300 calories and 30 grams of fat to your salad.

That's enough reason that salad dressing is a type of food to avoid for weight loss. To check how much fat and calories your salad dressing packs in, read labels. If you really can't seem to enjoy the taste of vinaigrette, which is a healthy option for a salad dressing, stick to using less salad dressing than what you normally would.

Regular Sodas

When you drink a 16oz glass of any regular soda, you take in about 197 calories more compared to diet soda of the same quantity. While you should skip drinking sodas altogether, if you can't just yet, try sticking to diet. Zero calories versus 197? You do the math.

Knowing which types of food to avoid for weight loss can be good for you. However, while these are the types of food to avoid for weight loss, it doesn't necessarily mean that you have to avoid them altogether.

Yes, it will be good for your body in the long run to avoid them all but they only really become harmful to you when you take them in excessive amounts.

If you really absolutely love these types of food to avoid for weight loss, try to indulge yourself every now and then. This will make you feel that you are not depriving yourself while at the same time not completely putting you off achieving your fitness goals.

If you have decided to indulge yourself in an effective weight loss program, it is necessary to put in all the required efforts to reach the success you yearn for. When you are fully focused on the specific weight loss plan you've designed, there may be some unwanted foods entering your diet that could lead to unpleasant results.

If you are not aware of your dietary habits, you could be eating foods that are reducing the progress instead of helping it. These foods could reverse the outcome expected from an effective weight loss program to a negative one.

CHAPTER 10
HABITS TO ADAPT YOUR BODY AGAINST WEIGHT GAIN

So to achieve your desired weight without sacrificing your daily lifestyle and health, I will give you the seven habits for highly effective Weight Loss Plan. These seven habits are highly required to adapt your body against weight gain which will help you learn the true essence of losing weight, naturally.

Here is the ultimate list of 7 habits for highly effective weight loss plan:

1. Eat healthy.

Eating a healthy diet for life will not only give you a healthier body but a fitter body as well. Eating more vegetables, fruits and other fiber-rich foods are crucial for your weight loss plan as these foods can burn fats easily.

The fiber content fills your stomach tightly, making you feel fuller all the time thus preventing unwanted snacking. The nutrients and vitamins that you will get from vegetables and fruits will also prevent you from developing dreaded diseases like heart disease and cancers.

2. Regular exercise

Regular exercise program is not new to us, but the problem is discipline. If you are not mentally prepared to do a fitness activity on a regular basis, you will certainly not going to lose those extra bulges on your belly.

Exercise comes on different forms and that's what makes this habit a fun one. Any physical activities such as dancing, sports, swimming, walking, jogging, cycling or even your normal morning car wash can all contributes to your exercise routine. So are you tired of having a regular exercise? You decide.

3. A daily dose of meditation

Meditation is a practice that helps relax the mind and body with powerful techniques. Once you focus on meditation, you also apply good posture that constitutes to a fine body figure.

Integrating mindfulness as one of your weight loss plan is a sure way to lose weight naturally without too much stress and financial expenditures. Truly, meditation is one sole practice that will not only give you health and wellness, but also Lose Weight potentials.

4. Avoid bad lifestyles

Lifestyles can either have negative or positive effects on our body, depending of course on your chosen habits. Bad lifestyles such as overconsumption of alcoholic beverages, smoking, illegal drug use, and many others, will inevitably cause your health to degrade and develop diseases.

What is more worse is that, it could lead to obesity as too much alcohol gives high concentration of calories especially beer. So whether you are on a weight loss plan or not, stay out of these bad vices to maintain good health and correct weight.

5. Be sociable and have fun

Did you know that a sociable person is more immune to weight gain? You are probably wondering how? Research concludes that being fun and sociable can develop the so called "brown fats" that helps lessen the white fats in the body.

White fat constitutes to weight gain while brown fat is usually found in babies. Through sociable interaction, brown fats can be developed and will add as your friendly Lose Weight buddy.

6. Control your cravings

This is one habit that you should successfully apply on your weight loss plan. All across our surroundings, there are different temptations that can lure us out of our weight loss plan.

There are sweet foods, junk foods, processed foods and many other products that can ultimately add up to our weight. Applying a strict discipline can give us the right course to weight loss success. Drive your mind into the right direction and you will certainly prevent weight gain.

7. Consult your physician, fitness expert or nutritionist

Consulting a fitness expert or a seasoned nutritionist will definitely help your weight loss endeavors. You can definitely depend on their advice as these people are an expert in the weight loss field. Make it a habit that you always visit your doctor for your weight loss concerns.

In summary, these seven habits for highly effective weight loss program can help you out of your weight gain dilemma. Keeping a healthy lifestyle plus a trusted weight loss habits can both overcome any types of weight loss issues.

The key to making effective weight loss decisions is to find a weight loss plan that you can use to maintain that weight loss for the rest of your life. Any diet which restricts your calorie intake to less than the calories your body is burning will work, short term.

The vast majority of diets are designed to do just that (work short term). To keep the weight off long-term, you have to exchange your unhealthy eating habits for healthy ones.

These new eating habits have to be incorporated into your life to the extent that you do them automatically. To work long term, you also have to incorporate at least a minimal amount of regular exercise into your life.

Diets that promise that you'll lose a large amount of weight quickly without changing your eating or exercise habits usually do not work at all unless the weight loss is caused by some sort of supplement such as diet pills or foods that raise your metabolic rate.

These types of diets usually claim that their pill or patch or fat blocker will give you miracle results. Some of these types of diets actually work but none of them work for the long term and most people start regaining the weight as soon as they stop taking the pill or eating the exact combination of foods, etc.

Low carb diets are very effective weight loss plans, especially for men, over the short term. Low carb (or high protein) diets work by restricting the amount of carbohydrates you are allowed to eat to under 10% (usually) and increasing the amount of protein and fat you consume (to 40% to 60%).

When you restrict carbohydrates, your body goes into a metabolic state called ketosis, where the body burns fat instead of carbs for fuel. Short term, this works great. Long term, however, this type of diet is believed to cause medical problems such as kidney failure, high cholesterol, kidney stones, gout, heart disease, and even osteoporosis.

Meal provider diets also work short term and are especially good for those dieters who lack the discipline (or the time) to follow less regimented diet plans. A meal provider diet is one in which most, or all, of your calorie restricted meals and snacks are delivered to you by the weight loss company.

Sometimes these meals are true meals and sometimes they are merely nutritional drinks/shakes or meal bars. Some of these types of diets are one-size-fits-all and some can be, at least somewhat, tailored to your likes and dislikes.

For a permanent solution to your weight problem you have to select a plan that you can adopt and maintain for life. Successful weight loss diets encourage permanent healthy changes to your eating and exercise habits.

Taking small baby steps and realizing this is a journey of a lifetime, not a sprint, will allow you make effective weight loss decisions and choose the right diet for you.

CHAPTER 12
LOSING WEIGHT AND GETTING SLIM IN JUST DAYS

Understand that fat is not going to just disappear. Let me make that clear right away. It is possible to lose some weight in a day, but not very much, and it is not a real fix for the fat that you are trying to get rid of.

In order for you to effectively get rid of the fat, you need your body to break it down and get rid of it. This is what happens when you expend more calories than you consume. The magic number is 3,500. That is roughly how many calories make up a pound. So how do you lose weight in a day?

When you hear people talking about losing 5, even 10 pounds in a day, first understand that what they did is not healthy. They more than likely did it one of 2 ways. The first way is by dropping water weight. This is often done with the help of pills, or some people use excessive exercise.

Wrestlers have been known to go running in a rubber suite, which seriously overheats the body, leading to excessive sweating. This is a very dangerous practice, and has been banned in most states for high school athletes. The second way that people often drop excessive weight □uickly is using laxatives. I'll let your imagination take over from there.

Why is it that people will neglect their health on a daily basis, but suddenly feel the need to lose some weight immediately for a special occasion. If you really care that much about what you look like, you need to make it something that you are aware of on a daily basis, as opposed to just on big days.

If you really want to know how to lose weight in a day, I cannot give you any healthy recommendations. If you have a week, or even better a month, then I can help you out.

Here are some tips for losing weight, in a healthy manner, in a short period of time.

1 - Yes, you need to exercise. When you are talking fitness, exercise is the king. If you are at all serious about losing weight, get started. It does not need to be anything crazy. The

more out of shape that you are, the faster you will typically get results....at least to a point. Start walking, riding a bike, something active.

2 - No more fast food. I know, it is super convenient and it tastes good. Which would you rather have, the 5 minutes of pleasure you get while eating the burger, or the ability to look in the mirror and feel good about yourself.

3 - Limit or eliminate soda from your diet. Again, I know, it is easy and it tastes good. Again, think about the long term effects.

4 - Get rid of the "how to lose weight in a day" mentality, and be consistent.

The best way to get your metabolic rate going is exercise, and plenty of it. The more exercise you do the more calories you burn and if you do fast walking or running you get an extra bonus of when you stop walking or running your body continues to burn calories for up to 4 hour afterwards.

With all that exercise you are doing, you will need to drink plenty of water. Now this is not to only to keep you hydrated when you are exercising. If you drink plenty of water your body will start to store less of it.

This means that you will carry less water weight. Another bonus of drinking lots of water is that it will help keep you full between meals so that you will feel the need to snack less.

Now moving onto meals, you will need to change your eating pattern so that you can lose as much weight as possible. But I stress... Don't follow the old fable of "eating less means losing weight." It just doesn't work like that. Our bodies are not designed to go without food. So if you start eating less, you will have the opposite effect of your intending result, meaning you will slow your metabolic rate down and store more fat.

So if you are going to lose weight you will need to eat more not less. Now I don't mean eat bigger meals, that's not going to work. What you are going to need to do is eat small meal regularly throughout the day. You will need at least 5 meals a day. Your body will see that it is getting enough food and it will start to burn all the calories you eat and more.

Daily Action Plan

If you want to lose weight in 10 days, it is best to have some sort of action plan lined up that you can work with day by day. I hope this procedure below will help you do just that and lose the most weight you can in 10 days in a safe manner.

So, what do your next 10 days need to look like? Let's see how you need to work out in order to achieve a safe and long term weight loss.

Day 1

On this day, you should do a strength and cardio workout. I recommend choosing 3 muscle groups and focusing on them in this workout session. The muscle groups are biceps, triceps, back, chest, shoulders, and legs. Don't do chest and back exercises together on the same workout.

At the end of the strength training, you need to do cardio. Make sure to make this cardio session intensive so you burn a lot of calories.

Day 2

On this day you should work the other 3 muscle groups with weights and do another cardio session.

Day 3

You don't need to go to the gym on this day but you may take a 30-45 minute walk in the evening in order to burn a bit more calories. You should also make sure to perform a long session of stretching exercises during this day.

Days 4, 7, 10

These days should be the same as day 1.

Day 5, 8

These days will have the same formation as day 2.

Day 6, 9

Days 6, 9 will be the same as Day 3.

Your workouts should be intensive. If you're not sweating and really feeling the effort, it means that you're not pushing yourself hard enough to lose the most weight in 10 days.

Nutrition

What you eat during these 10 days is also crucial for your success as you can't out train a bad diet. It will simply not work. Here are some tips for you to follow:

1. Don't drink alcohol. You can lay off the booze for 10 days. Alcohol is rich in calories and sugar and you don't need that when trying to shed weight.

2. Get rid of all sugary drinks and sodas. They're almost entirely devoid of nutritional benefits but full of calories.

3. Eat small meals throughout the day instead of 3 big ones. Don't skip meals as this can backfire and actually make you eat more.

4. Avoid fast food and pre-packaged dishes as these can often be full of sodium, sugar, and trans-fat. Always read labels before you buy food.

5. Eat lots of fruit and vegetables to help you get healthy sugar and have some good snacks ready.

Follow this advice and you may lose a lot of weight in 10 days.

CHAPTER 13
MINIMIZE SUGAR AND SODIUM INTAKE

Cutting back on one's sugar intake is a commonly discussed issue. High sugar levels in our bodies account for diabetes, and sugar is also associated with obesity and being overweight.

Alternately, sugar can have many negative effects on our health and wellbeing. It causes inflammation, and is known to induce erratic brain cell firing, wherein the communication between brain cells is altered. Sugar could even be addictive.

Excessive consumption of sugar has been linked with headaches, hypertension, fluid retention and even depression. But with the present day diet patterns, sometimes it could be tough to avoid excessive consumption of sugar.

A major portion of sugar consumption results not from our meals, but from the beverages that we have, and these may include coffee, alcoholic drinks, or even fruit juices.

As per a study conducted by the American Heart Association, on an average, American adults consume 22 teaspoons of sugar per day. And sugar consumption rates are higher still for teenagers in the United States. On an average, teenagers in the U.S consume 34 teaspoons of sugar per day.

But one can minimize sugar consumption without having to cut down on sweets. One must go for Stevia, a natural sweetener that has gained a great deal of prominence over the past few years. Stevia is a 100% natural sweetener.

And while it is 30 times sweeter than sugar, it has zero calories, zero carbohydrates, and has zero effect on our glycemic index. So it does not raise the insulin or blood sugar levels in our bodies at all.

Stevia is an herb. It is naturally sweet and is native to Paraguay. While Stevia is non-caloric, it has been used as a sweetener and even a flavor enhancer for centuries. Popularity of Stevia can further be highlighted by the fact that while Stevia finds more acceptance at all places in the world by the day, in Japan, around 40% of sweetener market is based on Stevia. So if one has sweet cravings, Stevia is undoubtedly the answer.

One of the facts that make Stevia all the more advantageous is that it is a 100% natural sweetener. If one chooses to go for artificial sweeteners, like in the form of diet sodas, these manipulate the body's ability to recognize how much one has eaten. So one tends to overeat without actually recognizing it.

There are many mechanisms by which Stevia works towards enabling us to avoid sugar. Stevia has zero sugar content, and so it ensures that cravings for sweet or fatty foods are reduced.

Additionally, being 100% herbal, Stevia keeps our body supple with nutrients. So one does not feel hunger pangs. Consuming Stevia in some form around 20 minutes before meals has been said to reduce hunger sensations.

Sodium

The importance of both salt and potassium in the diet was illustrated by a study - of almost 102,000 adults – which found that blood pressure levels are associated with both sodium and potassium intake. Sodium levels that are either too high or too low raise blood pressure, and high levels of potassium lower blood pressure.

The researchers concluded that an estimated intake of between 3 gram and 6g of salt (1.2g to 2.4g of sodium) a day was associated with a lower risk of cardiovascular events than either higher or lower levels. It also found that consumption of more than 1.5g of potassium a day was associated with a reduced risk of heart disease.

Sodium is an essential nutrient. However, because it retains excess fluids in the body, sodium increases blood pressure and so places an added burden on the heart.

If you are a type 2 diabetic, there is an 85% chance that you also have issues with your blood pressure. In addition, blood pressure tends to rise as you grow older.

Eating less sodium can help you control your blood pressure, which will reduce the risk that you develop stroke, heart failure, osteoporosis, stomach cancer, kidney disease and other associated medical conditions as time goes on.

But gaining control over the amount of sodium you eat can be difficult because about 75 percent of it comes from salt added to processed foods and restaurant foods. It's hard to limit your intake when the food you eat already contains lots of sodium.

Besides the sodium we ingest through salt added at the table or during cooking or the production of processed foods, there are several other sources of sodium in our diets.

Reading food labels you'll notice ingredients such as 'soda' (sodium bicarbonate, aka baking soda) and 'sodium' (in compounds such as sodium nitrate, sodium citrate, monosodium glutamate (MSG) and sodium benzoate). So you can get sodium in many foodstuffs, even those that don't taste salty.

It is estimated that, by 2020, nearly two-thirds of adults in the Western world will have high blood pressure due mainly to over-consumption of salt. Learning to read food labels is vital if you are to control your daily intake of sodium.

CHAPTER 14
THE IMPORTANCE OF KEEPING A WEIGHT LOSS JOURNAL

If you are really serious about losing weight, then there are a few things that you need to do to guarantee your success. One is eating right, another is exercise, but one of the most over looked parts is keeping a journal. Let's take a look at why journaling is so important.

As soon as you start a weight loss plan, you should start a journal. In the journal, you should record your starting weight, measurements and, if you have a scale to measure it, your body fat percentage.

You should also have a place to log in what you eat for each meal, any supplements you take to help your weight loss efforts, the type of exercise you are doing and the length of time you exercise.

Just the simple fact of having to log your eating and exercise habits will help keep you on track. It is hard to look at a blank page that was supposed to be completed and say, "I am eating right and exercising, but I cannot lose weight", right?

When you log your exercise, make sure you log the intensity of the exercise you are doing. For example, if you walk slowly or you walk at a fast pace. The amount of calories that will be burned will be greater at the faster pace. Having a record will allow you to adjust the amount and intensity of your exercise according to your fat loss results.

When you first start to exercise, you will not be as proficient and will be heavier which means you will burn more calories in the beginning. As you exercise more, you will get more mechanically proficient at the exercise and you will become lighter thus burning less calories for the same amount of exercise done.

For this reason, you will lose weight faster in the beginning and you may have to increase the intensity or length of time you exercise as you lose weight to see similar results.

By keeping good records in your journal, you will be able to adjust your routine in order to produce the results you desire. By recording what you eat, the amount and intensity of exercise, your weight and inches lost will give you a good foundation on which to base your adjustment decisions.

This will become your "weight loss diary" in the next coming weeks and you will rely heavily on it for guidance. Do not underestimate the power of keeping a weight loss journal. It is crucial to keep one for at least the first 12 weeks.

Think about the mental pressure you will place on yourself when you decide to skip exercise class or go grazing for chocolate cake and ice dream on the dessert bar when you know you must record what you ate and did not do at exercise class in the journal.

It will start to make you think twice before making a bad decision. Looking at your journal will keep you focused on your goal of being slimmer and fitting back into those tight, skinny, sexy jeans again.

When the weight does start to fall off and you can see written proof, it will give you inspiration to continue to lose more until you meet your weight loss goal. Set a target weight, record what you are doing in your journal and stick to it.

You may not see massive amounts of weight coming of in the beginning, but slowly and surely, the weight will come off and you will be able to see proof of pounds and inches gone in your journal.

You need not weigh everyday, but only once per week or every two weeks. As you follow your weight loss plan, you will start to notice your clothes fitting looser as inches start to melt away. This feeling, with the combination of physical proof from your journal, will keep you on track even through the hard times of temptation.

Keeping a journal is very important and is just one aspect of a complete weight loss plan. Make sure to include the journal in your complete plan to becoming slimmer and lighter.

CHAPTER 15
WEIGHT LOSS SUPPLEMENTS TO MAKE YOU STAY FIT

The single most common mistake people make while looking for fat loss supplements is that they go for chemically processed products that may work in the short run but over a period, the person becomes dependent on them to stay in shape.

In addition, most of these pills and processed chemical formulas alter the working of your heart and other body organs. So ultimately, they turn out to be unhealthy for the person's physical and general health.

Having said that, natural weight loss supplements for women do not have harmful effects. They assist our body to enhance its organs and circulatory system and metabolism to the extent that the body works more effectively without being hooked on external stimulants.

When evaluating weight loss supplements, perhaps you may encounter numerous pills and brands claiming to have 100 percent natural ingredients within their products. However, it is really not always the case; usually, the nature of the herbal product is changed completely by little processing and its benefits therefore are turned into secondary effects for the body.

Below are a few very effective natural weight loss supplements for women, which can help you shed much fat in a month. However, it should be noted here that all those natural supplements work as long as you keep a check on your diet and make your body used to some regular exercise whether either walking or exercising.

Natural or processed supplements alone cannot make a significant difference at the end. Let's look into those weight loss supplements.

Green Supplements:

These nutritional supplements can be obtained under different names and brand symbols. Green supplements usually comprise of small capsules that include extracts of just about thirty to thirty-six green leafy vegetables that help improve the metabolism of the body.

Initially, the diet plan supplement will surely have an opposite effect i.e. your craving for food might increase but after a number of days, the body adjusts to the properties of these capsules. Once adjusted, it cuts down on your appetite while increasing your metabolism, and as a result, you start burning the excess fat within your body.

Alkaline Supplements:

Alkaline vitamin supplements work by maintaining the acidity level of your system. They also come in the form of tablets, which will be consisting of natural products with high alkaline properties. These natural weight loss supplements for women affects the digestive system of the body; improving its efficiency and assisting you in digesting your meals ꞏuickly.

Furthermore, it makes you feel lighter and enhances your psychical activity. The sense of drowsiness and laziness reduces and you feel like going out and walking around on a regular basis. Because your rate of metabolism and muscle increase, you will start shedding weight without making any particular effort.

CHAPTER 16
POSITIVE WEIGHT LOSS AFFIRMATIONS

We gain weight in no time and again we have to adopt these same methods to reduce excess fats. Alternately, weight loss can be achieved through safe and natural way. The secret to achieve safe weight loss is through utilizing positive weight loss affirmations.

Positive weight loss affirmations act as a reprogramming software for the mind. They change your inner belief structure by implanting any thought, either positive or negative, into our minds in the form of a pattern when repeated many times.

Our subconscious then implements these pattern into our daily lives either leading to a positive or negative change. The reason that diet plans don't work well is that they may change your habits, but they rarely change your thought patterns.

Positive weight loss affirmations work the opposite way, changing your beliefs to achieve better habits. Coincidentally, using positive weight loss affirmations works far more effectively over the long term than simple diet plans alone.

The first step towards achieving your goal is to get rid of all those negative thoughts, inner-belief and behaviors which leads to weight problem in the first place such as 'I am so fat' or 'I am gaining weight every day'.

These thoughts hold you back from gaining an ideal weight. Your mind makes your body to gain weight since the mind is lead to believe that these negative thoughts are true. Start to lose weight by adopting a positive attitude. The more positive thoughts you have, the closer you are to slimming down.

Second step, and probably the most important one, is to live in the present. Instead of thinking about failures of the past, learn to live in the present and be determined to change what you could not achieve yesterday. Strengthen your self-image. Gain self-confidence. Believe in yourself and keep reminding yourself that you will lose weight or you feel lighter today. Build up your confidence as much as you can by going out in public places with the firm belief that you are one step closer to gaining your ideal weight and you are already succeeding.

This step involves implementing the beginnings of positive weight loss affirmations. By living and thinking in a way that presumes that you've already lost weight, your mind will begin to believe that it has already done so, making the process of actually losing weight with positive weight loss affirmations that much easier.

The wording you use is the key. You must use positive, simple and appropriate words for your mind to accept. You must truly believe whatever you say and then feel the emotions building up inside you.

You must get your mind to think that the positive weight loss affirmation you make can be made true. Never for one moment think 'can it happen?' Instead, think 'it can happen' or 'it is already happening'.

The positive weight loss affirmation needs to be repeated over many times in order for 'natural weight loss techni□ue' to succeed. You should write down any positive thought you have on a card and review them daily and most importantly first thing in the morning and before going to bed.

Some physiologists have recommended that if you have any negative thought write it down on a piece of paper. Later at the end of the day review it and try to come up with a more realistic positive statement. For example, instead of "I am so fat" you should think "I feel lighter today".

Whenever you think positive you are one step closer towards slimming and achieving your goal. Remember to create your own statement which your mind will actually believe to be true. Some examples of positive statement are given below:

I'm losing weight now.

I feel lighter today.

I love the feeling of making progress.

I love the food that makes me thin.

Losing weight is effortless.

I enjoy being healthy.

I'm feeling happy today.

My body is getting stronger, slimmer, and healthier every day.

CONCLUSION

The best diets for weight loss focus on making gradual lifestyle changes. Most people that experience significant amounts of weight gain do so when their eating habits veer from moderation towards excess. Learning to curb excessive eating and return to a more moderate and healthful lifestyle is typically the goal of any plan that will offer lasting benefits.

If you are looking to shed a few pounds in a hurry, than a crash diet can help you slim □uick. There is, however, a downside to dropping pounds at a super rapid speed. Most eating plans that severely cut calories also cut the amount of a nutrients that you intake.

This can be confusing to the body, which often responds by throwing itself into starvation mode. Your body interprets the sudden cessation of good eating as a sign of limited availability. In order to protect itself, the body then begins to ration calories and starts storing them as fat rather than burning them.

This is why many crash dieters find that even drastic changes in their eating habits will only have an effect for a short while. When the body is deprived, it begins to slow down. The weight drops off □uickly during the first few days of the crash diet, but in several weeks, it is hard to shed even a pound.

Crash diets are less than ideal, but they are also an effective way to drop a size or two in a hurry. These work well for shedding a few extra pounds before your wedding or vacation. The use of them should be limited however, because yo-yo dieting can ultimately be damaging to the metabolism and other body systems.

For many dieters, this is good news. Losing weight does not re□uire the total elimination of food groups nor does it have to mean suffering endless hours of stomach gurgling hunger pangs. In order to restore your physi□ue to its normal healthy size and measurements, you must simply restore normal and healthy habits of eating.

Staying properly hydrated is key for those who want to shed unwanted pounds. When the body is at a proper hydration level, most people find that they are far less prone to overeat.

One of the best things that you can do on any weight loss regimen is to start carrying a water body with you throughout the day and sipping wherever you go. You will find that not only do you naturally consume less when you do this, but you also feel better and have improved energy levels as well.

There are numerous diets for weight loss that can be found online today. You should work to find one that promotes a healthy, balanced and active lifestyle rather than one that requires long term cessation from the calories and nutrients that you need for optimal health. As a dieter, as you begin to exercise your body and your will power, you will find that both grow stronger each and every day.